Preface :

Working as a perfusionist is a h career path. The educational sta........... ... .g.., a.... ... profession appeals to those interested in working on surgical teams and in critical care scenarios.

Cardiac perfusion technology involves the use of medical devices and techniques to ensure that the heart is receiving sufficient blood flow and oxygenation. In emergency situations, errors can occur that can lead to serious complications, including heart failure and even death. Here are some common emergency scenarios and potential errors in cardiac perfusion technology. This book will help a Perfusionist to solve the problems in Cardiac Perfusion during Cardiac surgery and handle every emergency situation. To minimize the risk of errors and emergencies in cardiac perfusion technology, medical professionals must undergo extensive training in the use of perfusion machines and other equipment. They must also closely monitor patients during surgery and be prepared to intervene quickly in case of an emergency. Additionally, perfusion technology manufacturers must ensure that their machines meet strict safety standards and are regularly maintained to prevent malfunctions or defects. In this book we have explained the possible errors and emergency situations in a life of a Perfusionist. This complete solution book is made by the Perfusionist after years of experience and practical knowledge about the Perfusion techniques and skills required to be a quick problem solver.

Perfusion technology plays a crucial role in cardiovascular surgery, organ transplantation, and other medical procedures that require maintaining the oxygenation and circulation of vital organs. However, there are several challenges associated with perfusion technology that can impact patient outcomes. Addressing these challenges requires collaboration between healthcare providers, perfusionists, industry, and regulatory bodies to ensure safe, effective, and equitable delivery of perfusion technology to patients in need.

Perfusion technology is a vital component of cardiac surgery, and the role of perfusionists is crucial in ensuring patient safety and successful outcomes. By dedicating yourselves to learning more about perfusion technology, you are making a significant contribution to the field, and are demonstrating your commitment to the well-being of your patients.

I encourage you to continue your pursuit of knowledge and excellence in this field, and to stay engaged with the latest developments and best practices. By remaining curious, open-minded, and willing to learn, you can continue to grow and develop your skills as perfusionists, and make a meaningful impact in the lives of your patients.

Remember that every patient is unique, and every case presents its own challenges and opportunities. By staying focused, collaborative, and compassionate, you can help to ensure that your patients receive the highest quality of care, and achieve the best possible outcomes.

Thank you for your dedication to the field of perfusion technology, and for your commitment to improving patient care. Your efforts are truly appreciated, and I wish you all the best in your future endeavors.

TOPICS

1. Runaway Pump Head
2. Inadequate Venous Blood level return in reservior
3. Change Defective Oxygenator
4. Rupture of the pump head tube (PVC & SILOCON)
5. Massive Air Embolism
6. Water leak into Oxygenator
7. Hemotherm machine failure
8. Reverse connection of cannula to the Arterial and Venous line
9. Venous cannula partially dislodged
10. Aortic cannula in wrong position
11. Central oxygen supply failure
12. Distension of heart during CPB
13. Transfusion of Wrong unit of Blood
14. Protamine in CPB circuit
15. Power failure during CPB
16. Low level vortex in venous reservoir
17. Oxygen blender failure
18. Cardioplegia delivery system failure
19. Level sensor failure during CPB
20. Bubble detector failure

1. Runaway Pump Head

A cardiopulmonary perfusion pump is a medical device that helps support the circulation and oxygenation of a patient's blood during cardiac surgery or other procedures that require temporary circulatory support. The pump head is the component of the device that actually pumps the blood. "Runaway error" refers to a situation where the pump head is not functioning as intended and is running at an excessive or uncontrolled speed, which can result in serious harm or even death to the patient.

When a cardiopulmonary perfusion pump experiences a runaway error, it is crucial to quickly identify and correct the problem. This may involve checking the device's sensors and controls, replacing any faulty components, and recalibrating the pump head to ensure that it is operating within safe parameters.

In addition, medical staff should closely monitor the patient's vital signs and be prepared to take immediate action if their condition deteriorates. This may involve administering medications, adjusting the patient's ventilation, or even performing emergency surgery to address any complications that arise.

Overall, the key to managing a cardiopulmonary perfusion pump head runaway error is prompt detection, careful monitoring, and rapid intervention to ensure the safety and well-being of the patient.

Managing a cardiopulmonary perfusion pump runaway situation is a critical emergency that requires immediate attention from medical personnel. Here are some general steps that can be taken to manage this situation:

1. Stop the pump: The first step is to stop the pump immediately to prevent further damage or harm to the patient. Depending on the type of pump, this may involve flipping a switch or pressing a button.

2. Check the pump head: Once the pump is stopped, check the pump head for any visible signs of damage or malfunction. Inspect the tubing, connections, and any other components for signs of wear or damage that may have contributed to the runaway situation.

3. Check vital signs: Check the patient's vital signs, including heart rate, blood pressure, oxygen saturation, and other relevant metrics. Depending on the severity of the situation, medical personnel may need to take immediate action to stabilize the patient's condition.

4. Contact support: Contact the manufacturer's technical support or a qualified service provider to assist with troubleshooting and repairing the pump. They may be able to provide guidance on how to address the runaway situation, such as adjusting the pump head settings, replacing faulty components, or performing other maintenance tasks.

5. Consider alternative treatments: Depending on the severity of the situation and the availability of alternative treatment options, medical personnel may need to consider alternative treatments, such as manual perfusion, to provide circulatory support to the patient.

Important : FIRST STOP THE PUMP AND USE THE HAND CRANK TO RUN THE PUMP TO MAINTAIN THE ARTERIAL PRESSURE.

Of Hand Crank

In summary, managing a cardiopulmonary perfusion pump runaway situation requires a rapid and coordinated response from medical personnel. By stopping the pump, checking the pump head, monitoring the patient's vital signs, contacting technical support, and considering alternative treatments, medical personnel can work to ensure the safety and well-being of the patient.

2. Inadequate Venous Blood level return in reservior

Some possible causes of inadequate venous blood return in the cardiotomy reservoir include:

1. Cardiac tamponade: This occurs when blood accumulates around the heart, compressing it and reducing its ability to fill with blood.

2. Air embolism: Air can enter the circulatory system during surgery, blocking the flow of blood and reducing the amount of blood returning to the cardiotomy reservoir.

3. Vascular obstruction: Blood vessels in the surgical field may become blocked or compressed, reducing blood flow and causing inadequate venous blood return.

4. Pump malfunction: Malfunctions in the cardiopulmonary bypass pump or other equipment can result in inadequate blood flow and reduced venous blood return.

Low blood volume in the cardiotomy reservoir during cardiopulmonary bypass (CPB) can occur due to a number of factors, such as excessive blood loss during surgery or inadequate priming of the CPB circuit. Here are some general steps that can be taken to manage this situation:

1. Assess the situation: The first step is to assess the patient's vital signs and the blood flow through the CPB circuit. If the patient is showing signs of decreased cardiac output or hypotension, this may indicate a low blood volume in the cardiotomy reservoir.

2. Check the CPB circuit: Check the CPB circuit for any visible signs of leaks, kinks, or other obstructions that may be impeding the flow of blood. Also check the cardiotomy reservoir for proper filling and drainage.

3. Increase flow rate: If the flow rate through the CPB circuit is low, increasing the flow rate of the bypass pump may help increase blood volume in the cardiotomy reservoir. This can be done gradually, while monitoring the patient's vital signs to avoid potential complications.

4. Administer fluids: Administering fluids, such as crystalloids or colloids, can help increase the volume of blood in the cardiotomy reservoir. The type and amount of fluids administered will depend on the patient's individual needs and the underlying cause of the low blood volume.

5. Transfuse blood products: If the low blood volume is due to excessive blood loss, transfusing blood products such as packed red blood cells or fresh frozen plasma may be necessary to replace the lost blood volume.

6. Consider additional interventions: In some cases, additional interventions may be necessary to address the underlying cause of the low blood volume, such as repairing a vascular injury or addressing a coagulation disorder.

In summary, managing low blood volume in the cardiotomy reservoir during cardiopulmonary bypass requires a thorough assessment of the patient's condition, careful monitoring of vital signs, and prompt intervention to address the underlying cause of the problem. By increasing the flow rate, administering fluids, transfusing blood products, and considering additional interventions as necessary, medical personnel can work to restore the patient's blood volume and ensure the best possible outcome.

3. Change Defective Oxygenator

Changing a defective oxygenator during cardiopulmonary bypass (CPB) requires careful planning and execution to minimize the risk of complications. Here are the general steps involved in changing a defective oxygenator during CPB.

Reasons of oxygenator replacement:

1. Low oxygenation
It can be detected by dark coloured arterial blood. Cross-check the blood gas samples irrespective of the 100% oxygen flow to the oxygenator.

2. Leaking oxygenator.

3. High inlet pressure which restricts the adequacy of perfusion.

4. clot formation in the oxygenator.

Procedure to change the oxygenator:

1. Notify the surgeon and anaesthesiologist of the problem. Seek required assistance.

2. Initiate cooling of the patient and administer cerebroprotective drugs if required.

3. Open the replacement oxygenator and keep ready.

4. come off bypass and clamp the inlet and outlet of the oxygenator with two clamps on each side. Cut the inlet tube in between the gap of the two clamps. Then cut the outlet tube in between the two clamps.

5. Connect the oxygen line to the oxygenator.

6. Connect the inlet and outlet to the replacement oxygenator and connect the recirculating line of the replacement oxygenator to the reservoir. Connect the sampling ports. Remove the clamps on inlet and outlet then clamp the aortic line. Open the recirculating line and de-air the oxygenator.

7.Stop the arterial pump and clamp the recirculating line after de-airing the oxygenator.

8. Notify the surgeon CPB is ready to go on.

9. Fix the replacement oxygenator in the stand. Remove clamps on arterial line and restart CBP. Keep the oxygen supply on.

In summary, changing a defective oxygenator during cardiopulmonary bypass requires careful coordination and execution to ensure that the patient's condition remains stable and that the procedure is performed safely and effectively. By following the appropriate steps and closely monitoring the patient throughout the process, medical personnel can help minimize the risk of complications and ensure the best possible outcome.

4. Rupture of the pump head tube (PVC & SILOCON)

A ruptured arterial PVC tube during cardiopulmonary bypass (CPB) is a serious situation that requires immediate action to prevent the patient from losing blood and experiencing severe hypotension. Here are the general steps involved in managing this situation.

1. Notify the surgical team: Alert the surgical team immediately of the ruptured PVC tube, and coordinate with them to ensure that the necessary equipment and personnel are available.

2. Stop the blood flow: Stop the blood flow through the CPB circuit immediately to minimize blood loss.

3. Clamp the affected line: Clamp the affected arterial line to prevent further blood loss.

4. Assess the situation: Assess the patient's condition, vital signs, and the extent of the bleeding.

5. Replace the ruptured PVC tube: Replace the ruptured PVC tube with a new one, making sure that all connections are secure and free from air bubbles.

6. Restart the blood flow: Restart the blood flow through the CPB circuit and adjust the flow rate as needed.

7. Monitor the patient: Closely monitor the patient's vital signs and watch for any signs of complications, such as bleeding or hypotension.

8. Post-operative care: After the procedure, closely monitor the patient's vital signs and watch for any signs of complications, such as bleeding or thrombosis.

5. Massive Air Embolism

Air embolism during cardiopulmonary bypass (CPB) is a rare but potentially life-threatening complication. Management of massive air embolism during CPB requires prompt recognition and immediate intervention. Here are some steps that can be taken:

1. Stop the CPB pump immediately: The first step is to stop the CPB pump to prevent further air from entering the patient's circulation.

2. Position the patient: Place the patient in a left lateral decubitus position with the head down to trap the air in the right ventricle and prevent it from entering the pulmonary artery.

3. Aspirate air: Use a large-bore central venous catheter or a right heart catheter to aspirate air from the right atrium, superior vena cava, and pulmonary artery. This will help to remove the air from the circulation.

4. Administer oxygen: Administer 100% oxygen to the patient to displace the air in the lungs and improve oxygenation.

5. Initiate cardiopulmonary resuscitation (CPR): If the patient becomes hemodynamically unstable, initiate CPR and consider defibrillation if the patient develops a cardiac arrest.

6. Provide supportive care: Provide supportive care including volume resuscitation, inotropes, and vasopressors to maintain blood pressure and organ perfusion.

7. Identify the source of air: Identify the source of the air embolism and take appropriate steps to prevent it from recurring.

8. Place the patient in steep Trendelenburg's position (Head down position)

9. Clamp venous line & open recirculating line and allow bubbles in arteria line to passively retrogradely drain by gravity.

10. For small air bubbles in arterial line the surgeon removes A-line cannula, flush blood , for large bubbles the surgeon joins A-line to V-line, recirculate and prime circuit.

11. Re-establish antegrade CPB. Hypeothermia 20*C to increase gas bubble solubility, minimise organ damage due to hypoperfusion.

12. induce hypertension - Vasoconstrictor drugs

13. Remove coronary air by massaging & needle venting.

14. Drugs - Steriods, Manitol. Perfusion for45 min. Wean off CPB

Retrograde Cerebral Perfusion

1. Connect arterial line to SVC cannula with tourniquet. Perfuse 20*C blood into SVC, measuring cerebral pressure from internal jugular (< 25 mmHg).

2. Coronary sinus cannula in SVC - Perfusion 20*C blood at 600 ml/ml via coronary sinus, measuring cerebral pressure (< 25 mmHg).

3. Air + Blood drain from the aortic cannula. Carotid compression is performed.

4. Continue for 5 minutes after air is seen exiting aorta.

6. Water leak into Oxygenator

Water leakage into the oxygenator from the heat exchanger during cardiopulmonary perfusion is a serious issue that can lead to hypoxemia and hemodynamic instability. Management of this problem requires quick action to prevent any harm to the patient. Here are some steps that can be taken.

1. Stop the perfusion pump immediately: The first step is to stop the perfusion pump to prevent further water from entering the oxygenator and the patient's circulation.
2. Check the source of the leak: Identify the source of the water leak and isolate the heat exchanger to prevent further water leakage.

3. Replace the oxygenator: If the oxygenator has been contaminated by water, it must be replaced immediately.

4. Administer 100% oxygen: Administer 100% oxygen to the patient to improve oxygenation.

5. Provide supportive care: Provide supportive care including volume resuscitation, inotropes, and vasopressors to maintain blood pressure and organ perfusion.

6. Monitor the patient closely: Monitor the patient's vital signs, arterial blood gases, and oxygen saturation closely to detect any changes in the patient's condition.

7. Consider ECMO: In severe cases, extracorporeal membrane oxygenation (ECMO) may be considered to support the patient's oxygenation and circulation while the issue is being addressed.

Prevention : Check the heat exchanger by circulating water before the oxygenator. Observe for a raising fluid level in the oxygenator.

Diagnosis :

• Rising venous reservoir water level without addition of fluid.

• sudden Haemodilution, Haemoglobinuria

• Dropped saturation.

Management:

• Stop Hemotherm machine immediately. Change the defective oxygenator.

• Administer antibiotics and diuretics.

• Use hemp filters or cell savers and add blood.

• increase FiO2 100%

In summary, managing water leakage into the oxygenator from the heat exchanger during cardiopulmonary perfusion requires quick action to stop the perfusion pump, identify the source of the leak, replace the oxygenator if necessary, administer 100% oxygen, provide supportive care, monitor the patient closely, and consider ECMO if necessary. Early intervention can prevent serious complications and improve patient outcomes.

7. Hemotherm machine failure

Hemotherm machine failure during cardiopulmonary perfusion can lead to hypothermia or hyperthermia, which can have serious consequences for the patient. Here are some steps that can be taken to manage Hemotherm machine failure:

1. Use external warmers to keep the patient warm or use ice pack around the patient and oxygenator to cool the patient at certain levels.

2. Check the Hemotherm machine: Check the Hemotherm machine for any malfunctions or errors and attempt to correct the problem. If the problem cannot be corrected quickly, switch to a backup machine if available.

3. Monitor the patient's temperature: Monitor the patient's temperature closely and take appropriate measures to maintain normothermia. If the patient is hypothermic, use warm blankets, heated humidified gases, and warm intravenous fluids to rewarm the patient. If the patient is hyperthermic, use cooling blankets or ice packs, and provide cold fluids to cool the patient.

4. Adjust the perfusion flow rate: Adjust the perfusion flow rate to maintain adequate organ perfusion and oxygenation.

5. Administer medications: Administer medications as needed to control the patient's blood pressure, heart rate, and arrhythmias.

6. Consider ECMO: In severe cases, extracorporeal membrane oxygenation (ECMO) may be considered to support the patient's circulation while the Hemotherm machine is being repaired or replaced.

7. Notify the surgical team: Notify the surgical team of the situation and keep them informed of the patient's condition.

Warming patient with hemotherm machine :

Maintaining normothermia is crucial during cardiopulmonary perfusion to prevent hypothermia and its associated complications. If the Hemotherm machine fails or is not available, there are several methods to warm the patient during cardiopulmonary perfusion:

1. Warm blankets: Use warm blankets to cover the patient to reduce heat loss from the skin surface. The blankets should be pre-warmed before use.

2. Heated humidified gases: Use heated and humidified gases such as oxygen to warm the patient's airway and lungs.

3. Warm intravenous fluids: Administer warmed intravenous fluids to the patient to maintain core body temperature.

4. Forced air warming: Use forced air warming devices such as Bair Hugger or Warm Touch to warm the patient.

5. Warm water blankets: Use warm water blankets to cover the patient's torso and limbs to reduce heat loss from the skin surface.

6. Active warming devices: Use active warming devices such as warming pads or mattresses that are designed to warm the patient.

7. Warm irrigation solution: Use warm irrigation solution during surgery to warm the patient from within.

In summary, there are several methods to warm the patient during cardiopulmonary perfusion if the Hemotherm machine fails or is not available. These methods include warm blankets, heated humidified gases, warm intravenous fluids, forced air warming, warm water blankets, active warming devices, and warm irrigation solution.

8. Reverse connection of cannula to the Arterial and Venous line

Reversal of the arterial and venous lines to the cannula during cardiopulmonary bypass is a potentially life-threatening complication that must be addressed immediately. The following steps can be taken to manage this situation:

1. Stop the cardiopulmonary bypass machine immediately to prevent further damage.

2. Notify the perfusionist, surgeon, and anesthesia team of the reversal of lines.

3. Clamp the arterial line as close to the cannula as possible to prevent oxygenated blood from flowing to the venous side.

4. Unclamp the venous line to allow deoxygenated blood to flow to the oxygenator.

5. Reverse the lines to the correct position by disconnecting them from the cannula and reattaching them in the proper position.

6. Check for air in the lines and remove it by purging the system.
Restart the cardiopulmonary bypass machine and slowly resume flow, monitoring for any signs of hemodynamic instability or gas exchange abnormalities.

7. Inform the surgical team of any potential complications, and consider performing additional monitoring and testing to ensure that the patient is stable.

It is crucial to act quickly and efficiently to reverse the lines and prevent further damage to the patient. Perfusionists and other members of the surgical team should be trained to recognize and respond to this complication promptly.

9. Venous cannula partially dislodged

A partially dislodged venous cannula during cardiopulmonary bypass can lead to decreased venous return and decreased oxygenation of the patient. The following steps can be taken to manage this situation:

1. Stop the cardiopulmonary bypass machine immediately to prevent further damage.

2. Notify the perfusionist, surgeon, and anesthesia team of the partially dislodged venous cannula.

3. Check the position of the venous cannula by visual inspection and palpation to determine the degree of displacement.

4. If the cannula is only partially dislodged and the blood flow is not compromised, it may be repositioned gently by rotating it in the correct direction.

5. If the cannula is severely dislodged and the blood flow is compromised, clamp the venous line to prevent air entry into the system, which can cause an air embolism.

6. Reposition the cannula by gently guiding it back into the correct position.

7. Check for air in the lines and remove it by purging the system

8. Restart the cardiopulmonary bypass machine and slowly resume flow, monitoring for any signs of hemodynamic instability or gas exchange abnormalities.

9. Inform the surgical team of any potential complications and consider performing additional monitoring and testing to ensure that the patient is stable.

10. Aortic cannula in wrong position

The malposition of an aortic cannula during cardiopulmonary bypass can lead to inadequate perfusion and oxygenation of the patient. Here are some ways to detect the malposition of an aortic cannula:

1. Inspect the position of the aortic cannula - During the bypass procedure, a perfusionist or surgeon should be continuously monitoring the position of the cannula to ensure that it is in the correct position. If the position appears to be off, then further investigation is required.

2. Assess blood flow - The perfusionist should monitor the blood flow through the aortic cannula. If there is a significant reduction in the flow, it may be an indicator of a malpositioned cannula.

3. Assess oxygen saturation - A decrease in oxygen saturation can indicate that the aortic cannula is not in the correct position.

4. Monitor arterial pressure - A decrease in arterial pressure can also indicate that the aortic cannula is not in the correct position.

5. Use imaging techniques - Ultrasound or fluoroscopy can be used to visualize the position of the cannula.

6. Confirm position of the aortic cannula - A perfusionist or surgeon can confirm the position of the aortic cannula by visual inspection and palpation.

It is important to detect the malposition of the aortic cannula as soon as possible to prevent complications such as cerebral ischemia, renal failure, or other organ damage. In addition, proper training and regular assessment of the perfusionist and surgical team can help prevent such complications from occurring.

Malposition of the aortic cannula during cardiopulmonary bypass can lead to inadequate perfusion and oxygenation of the patient. The following steps can be taken to manage this situation:

1. Stop the cardiopulmonary bypass machine immediately to prevent further damage.

2. Notify the perfusionist, surgeon, and anesthesia team of the malpositioned aortic cannula.

3. Check the position of the aortic cannula by visual inspection and palpation to determine the degree of displacement.

4. the cannula is only slightly malpositioned and the blood flow is not compromised, it may be repositioned gently by rotating it in the correct direction.

5. If the cannula is significantly malpositioned and the blood flow is compromised, clamp the aortic line to prevent air entry into the system, which can cause an air embolism.

6. Reposition the aortic cannula by gently guiding it back into the correct position.

7. Check for air in the lines and remove it by purging the system.

8. Restart the cardiopulmonary bypass machine and slowly resume flow, monitoring for any signs of hemodynamic instability or gas exchange abnormalities.

9. inform the surgical team of any potential complications and consider performing additional monitoring and testing to ensure that the patient is stable.

If the aortic cannula cannot be repositioned, it may be necessary to replace it with a new cannula.

11. Central oxygen supply failure

In the event of a central oxygen supply failure during cardiopulmonary bypass, the following steps should be taken:

1. Notify the perfusionist and surgical team immediately.

2. Switch to the backup oxygen supply, such as a portable tank, if available.

3. a backup oxygen supply is not available, manually ventilate the patient using a bag-valve-mask ventilation device.

4. Monitor the patient's oxygen saturation levels and blood gases closely to ensure adequate oxygenation.

5. Assess the oxygen demand of the patient and adjust the oxygen flow rate accordingly.

6. Consider alternative methods of oxygenation, such as extracorporeal membrane oxygenation (ECMO), if the backup supply or manual ventilation is insufficient to meet the patient's oxygen demand.

7. Inform the hospital's facilities management team to investigate the cause of the central oxygen supply failure and restore the supply as soon as possible.

It is essential to act quickly to ensure the patient's safety and prevent complications such as hypoxia, ischemia, or brain damage. Additionally, the surgical team should be prepared to manage such emergencies, and the perfusionist should regularly check the oxygen supply and ensure that backup supplies are available and functioning properly.

12. Distension of heart during CPB

Distension of the heart during cardiopulmonary bypass (CPB) can occur due to various factors such as improper drainage, over-perfusion, or ventricular dysfunction. The following steps should be taken to manage distension of the heart during CPB:

1. Notify the perfusionist and surgical team immediately.

2. Assess the cause of heart distension, including monitoring the central venous pressure (CVP), pulmonary artery pressure (PAP), and cardiac output (CO).

3. Reduce the pump flow rate or adjust the venous drainage to decrease the volume of blood returning to the heart.

4. Administer medications such as diuretics, inotropes, or vasodilators to reduce the volume of blood in the heart and improve cardiac function.

5. Consider using a left ventricular vent to drain blood from the left ventricle to reduce the pressure in the heart.

6. Perform an intraoperative echocardiogram to assess the cardiac function and determine the cause of the heart distension.

7. If the heart distension is due to ventricular dysfunction, consider administering medications such as milrinone, dobutamine, or epinephrine to improve cardiac contractility

8. Monitor the patient's vital signs, including blood pressure, heart rate, and oxygen saturation, closely to assess the effectiveness of the intervention.

It is essential to act quickly to prevent further complications such as pulmonary edema, decreased cardiac output, or even cardiac arrest.

13. Transfusion of Wrong unit of Blood

The transfusion of the wrong unit of blood during cardiopulmonary bypass can be a serious medical error that may lead to severe complications and even death. Therefore, it is important to have a protocol in place to manage such incidents. Here are some steps that can be taken:

1. Stop the transfusion immediately: If a transfusion of the wrong unit of blood is identified during cardiopulmonary bypass, the first step is to stop the transfusion immediately.

2. The medical team should be notified immediately so that they can take appropriate action. This may include consulting with a hematologist or blood bank specialist to determine the extent of the problem and the necessary steps to take.

3. Identify the patient and donor units: The patient and donor units should be identified to determine the extent of the mismatch. This can be done by checking the labels on the bags or the barcodes on the units.

4. Assess the patient's condition: The patient's condition should be assessed to determine the extent of the damage caused by the mismatch. This may include checking vital signs, performing laboratory tests, and assessing for signs of hemolysis or other complications.

5. Provide appropriate treatment: Depending on the severity of the mismatch and the patient's condition, appropriate treatment should be provided. This may include stopping the transfusion, administering medications to treat any complications, or providing supportive care.

6. Report the incident: The incident should be reported to the appropriate authorities, such as the hospital's quality control department or regulatory agencies. This can help prevent similar incidents in the future and ensure that appropriate action is taken to address the problem.

Preventing wrong transfusion of blood unit during cardiopulmonary bypass is crucial for patient safety. Here are some steps that can be taken to avoid such errors:

1. Proper identification of the patient: The patient's identity should be verified using at least two identifiers, such as name, date of birth, and medical record number.

2. Proper identification of the blood unit: The blood unit should be properly labeled with the patient's name and identification number to ensure that it is intended for that patient.

3. Use of barcoding technology: Barcoding technology can be used to verify the blood unit and ensure that it matches the patient's identification.

4. Verification by two qualified personnel: The blood unit should be verified by at least two qualified personnel, such as a nurse and a technician, before it is administered to the patient.

5. Standardized procedures and checklists: Standardized procedures and checklists can be used to ensure that all steps of the transfusion process are followed correctly.

6. Proper training and education: Healthcare professionals involved in the transfusion process should receive proper training and education on the procedures and protocols for safe blood transfusion.

7. Use of transfusion management systems: Transfusion management systems can be used to track and monitor the transfusion process and provide alerts if there is a mismatch between the patient and the blood unit.

14. Protamine in CPB circuit

If protamine gets into the oxygenator during cardiopulmonary bypass (CPB), Here are some steps that can be taken to manage protamine in the oxygenator during CPB:

1. If protamine is identified in the oxygenator, the infusion should be stopped immediately to prevent further damage to the membrane.

2. Check for oxygenator integrity: The integrity of the oxygenator should be checked to determine the extent of the damage caused by the protamine. This may include checking for leaks or discoloration of the membrane.

3. The patient's condition should be assessed to determine the extent of the hypoxemia caused by the protamine. This may include checking vital signs, blood gas levels, and assessing for signs of organ dysfunction.

4. Depending on the severity of the hypoxemia, appropriate treatment should be provided. This may include administering oxygen or other supportive measures, such as heparin to avoid clotting.

5. If the damage to the oxygenator is significant, it may need to be replaced. This can be done during the CPB procedure if necessary.

6. The incident should be reported to the appropriate authorities, such as the hospital's quality control department or regulatory agencies. This can help prevent similar incidents in the future and ensure that appropriate action is taken to address the problem.

7. A root cause analysis should be conducted to determine the underlying causes of the incident and identify areas for improvement in the CPB process.

15. Power failure during CPB

A power failure during cardiopulmonary bypass (CPB) can be a life-threatening emergency. Here are some steps that can be taken to manage a power failure during CPB:

1. Notify the surgical team: If the power failure is detected, the surgical team should be notified immediately. This can help them prepare to manage the situation and ensure that the patient remains safe.

2. Initiate emergency backup power: Most hospitals have backup power systems that can be activated in the event of a power failure. These systems typically include emergency generators or uninterruptible power supplies (UPS) that can provide power to critical equipment such as the CPB machine and monitors.

3. Check the CPB machine: Once backup power is activated, the CPB machine should be checked to ensure that it is functioning properly. This may include checking the battery backup systems, making sure the flow rates are appropriate, and ensuring that the alarms are functioning properly.

4. Check the patient's condition: The patient's condition should be monitored closely to ensure that there are no adverse effects of the power failure.

5. The hospital administration should be notified of the power failure and steps taken to manage the situation. This can help ensure that appropriate resources and support are available to manage the emergency.

6. Once the power is restored and the emergency is resolved, a post-incident analysis should be conducted to determine the root cause of the power failure and identify areas for improvement in the hospital's emergency preparedness plan.

7. Use the hand crank to continue Perfusion till the issue is resolved.

16. Low level vortex in venous reservoir

Low-level vortex in the venous reservoir during cardiopulmonary bypass (CPB) can lead to the entrainment of air and the formation of microbubbles, which can cause significant complications such as systemic embolization and gas embolism. Here are some strategies to manage low-level vortex in the venous reservoir during CPB:

1. Adjust the level of blood in the venous reservoir: Ensuring that the level of blood in the venous reservoir is sufficient can help reduce the formation of vortexes. The blood level should be maintained between the upper and lower level lines indicated on the reservoir.

2. Proper placement and positioning of the venous cannula can help reduce the formation of vortexes in the venous reservoir. The cannula should be placed in the superior vena cava, and the tip should be positioned near the right atrium.

3. Use of filters: Installing an in-line filter in the venous line can help prevent the formation of vortexes and the entrainment of air. The filter should be checked regularly and changed as needed.

4. Minimizing turbulence: Minimizing turbulence in the venous reservoir can help reduce the risk of vortex formation. This can be achieved by ensuring the venous line is properly secured, avoiding kinks or bends in the line, and maintaining proper flow rates.

5. Use of antifoam agents: Adding an antifoam agent, such as polydimethylsiloxane, to the venous reservoir can help reduce the formation of vortexes and the entrainment of air.

6. Monitoring: Regular monitoring of the venous reservoir during CPB can help detect any vortex formation or entrainment of air. Immediate action can be taken to prevent further complications..

17. Oxygen blender failure

Oxygen blender failure on the heart-lung machine during cardiopulmonary bypass (CPB) can lead to hypoxemia and other serious complications. Here are some strategies to manage oxygen blender failure during CPB:

1. Check the oxygen flow: The first step in managing oxygen blender failure is to check the oxygen flow to the oxygenator. If the oxygen flow is low or absent, the oxygen supply should be checked and corrected as necessary.

2. Use backup oxygen sources: The heart-lung machine should be equipped with backup oxygen sources, such as portable oxygen cylinders or a backup oxygen blender. These should be used immediately if the primary oxygen blender fails.

3. Increase the FiO2: If the oxygen blender failure cannot be corrected, the fraction of inspired oxygen (FiO2) delivered to the patient can be increased manually to maintain adequate oxygenation. This can be done by increasing the oxygen flow or adjusting the oxygen concentration on the backup blender

4. Monitor oxygen saturation: Continuous monitoring of oxygen saturation is essential to detect hypoxemia early. The oxygen saturation should be monitored using pulse oximetry or arterial blood gas analysis.

5. Consider alternative oxygenation strategies: If hypoxemia cannot be corrected by increasing the FiO2, alternative oxygenation strategies, such as extracorporeal membrane oxygenation (ECMO) or partial bypass, may be necessary.

6. Notify the surgical team: In the event of oxygen blender failure, the surgical team should be notified immediately so that appropriate interventions can be made.

Prompt recognition and management of oxygen blender failure is essential to prevent hypoxemia and other serious complications.

18. Cardioplegia delivery system failure

Cardioplegia delivery system leaking during cardiopulmonary bypass (CPB) can lead to inadequate cardiac protection and compromise the success of the surgery. Here are some strategies to manage cardioplegia delivery system leaking during CPB:

1. Identify the source of the leak: The first step in managing cardioplegia delivery system leaking is to identify the source of the leak. This can be done by visually inspecting the cardioplegia delivery system for any signs of damage or leakage.

2. Replace or repair damaged components: If the source of the leak is identified, the damaged components should be replaced or repaired as soon as possible. This can include replacing faulty tubing or connectors, or repairing any tears or holes in the cardioplegia device.

3. Use alternative cardioplegia delivery system: If the leak cannot be repaired immediately, an alternative cardioplegia delivery system can be used. This may include a different delivery system or the use of an alternative route.

4. Monitor myocardial protection: In the event of a leak, it is important to closely monitor myocardial protection to ensure that adequate cardioplegia is delivered. This can be done by monitoring cardiac function, such as electrocardiogram (ECG) changes, and measuring the levels of potassium in the blood.

5. Notify the surgical team: The surgical team should be notified immediately of any cardioplegia delivery system leaks. They may need to adjust the surgical plan or take additional measures to ensure adequate myocardial protection.

6. Document the incident: Any incidents of cardioplegia delivery system leaking should be documented in the patient's medical record for future reference.

19. Level sensor failure during CPB

Level sensor failure during cardiopulmonary bypass (CPB) can lead to inadequate fluid management and potential patient harm. Here are some strategies to manage level sensor failure during CPB:

1. Check fluid levels manually: The first step in managing level sensor failure is to check fluid levels manually. This can be done by visually inspecting the fluid levels in the reservoirs or using a dipstick to measure the fluid levels.

2. Use backup level sensors: The heart-lung machine should be equipped with backup level sensors, which can be used in the event of sensor failure. The backup sensors should be calibrated and tested regularly to ensure their accuracy.

3. Monitor fluid balance: In the event of level sensor failure, it is important to monitor fluid balance closely to prevent fluid overload or depletion. This can be done by monitoring urine output, blood pressure, and other relevant clinical parameters.

4. Adjust flow rates: If the level sensor failure cannot be corrected, the flow rates can be adjusted manually to maintain the desired fluid balance. This may require adjusting the pump speeds or manually regulating the fluid flow.

5. Notify the surgical team: The surgical team should be notified immediately of any level sensor failures so that appropriate interventions can be made.

6. Document the incident: Any incidents of level sensor failure should be documented in the patient's medical record for future reference.

20. Bubble detector failure

Bubbles detector failure during cardiopulmonary bypass (CPB) can lead to the potential for air embolism and other complications. Here are some strategies to manage bubbles detector failure during CPB:

1. Use alternative methods for detecting bubbles: In the event of bubbles detector failure, alternative methods for detecting bubbles can be used. These may include visual inspection of the venous and arterial lines for air, or the use of other bubble detectors if available.

2. Monitor the patient closely: In the event of bubbles detector failure, the patient should be monitored closely post opp for signs of air embolism, such as changes in mental status, seizures, or respiratory distress. Vital signs, such as blood pressure, heart rate, and oxygen saturation, should also be closely monitored.

3. Notify the surgical team: The surgical team should be notified immediately of any bubbles detector failures or suspected air embolism. They may need to adjust the surgical plan or take additional measures to ensure patient safety.

4. Document the incident: Any incidents of bubbles detector failure or suspected air embolism should be documented in the patient's medical record for future reference.

5. Inspect the circuit regularly: The CPB circuit should be inspected regularly during CPB to ensure that there are no air leaks or other sources of bubbles.

In summary, avoiding bubbles in the CPB circuit during CPB requires proper priming, minimizing turbulence, using air eliminators, inspecting the circuit regularly.

Dear readers,

I want to express my heartfelt gratitude for your interest and support of the perfusion technology book that I have written. I am truly honored to have had the opportunity to share my knowledge and experience with you.

It is my sincere hope that the information presented in the book has been helpful in advancing your understanding of perfusion technology, and has provided practical guidance on the use of cardiopulmonary bypass and other essential techniques in cardiac surgery. I have worked hard to ensure that the book is comprehensive, up-to-date, and accessible to a wide range of healthcare professionals involved in perfusion technology.

Your feedback and engagement is crucial to the success of this book, and I am grateful for your support. I hope that it will continue to serve as a valuable resource for you, and that it will contribute to improving patient outcomes and advancing the field of cardiac surgery.

Once again, thank you for your interest in this book, and for your dedication to improving healthcare through the use of perfusion technology.

Sincerely,

Vivek .V. Paul
(Cardiac Perfusionist)